THE DASH DIET MEAL PREP FOR SENIORS

Easy to make recipes to balance blood level and boost vitality

JORDAN MARGUIRE

Jordan Marguire

TABLE OF CONTENTS

FORWARD

Introducing the Dash Diet Meal Prep Cookbook, designed specifically for seniors looking to use food to boost their energy, control their blood pressure, and enhance their health. While being older is a beautiful journey filled with experiences and wisdom, it also commonly results in the emergence of new health problems. This cookbook serves as a guide for seniors to adopt the popular Dash Diet ideals and take control of their health. It's more than just a collection of recipes. As we become older, our bodies require a more thoughtful approach to eating. Dietary Approaches to Stop Hypertension, sometimes known as the Dash Diet, has received international recognition for its ability to effectively reduce blood pressure, improve heart health, and promote overall wellness. In this cookbook, we've adjusted these ideas to suit the requirements and preferences of elderly citizens.

These pages provide thoughtfully crafted, delectable, simple, and quick-to-follow recipes. They ensure that every meal not only supports optimal health but also satisfies the palate. They are an ode to flavor, health, and usefulness. Why focus on cooking? Since we understand the value of convenience without compromising one's health. You may save time and work and ensure that a week's worth of nutritious, well-balanced meals is always available by planning your cooking.

Achieving blood level balance and boosting vitality are practical goals, not pipe dreams. You may embark on a journey that celebrates delectable food, promotes physical health, and offers you a new lease on life with the aid of this cookbook. Whether you're a novice or an expert chef, this cookbook is your culinary companion. This is the ideal time to rekindle your love of cooking and use each meal to nurture your body and soul.

Join us as we explore a world of flavors, wholesome meals, and the transforming power of the Dash Diet Meal Prep Cookbook for Seniors. Let's toast to your health, pleasure, and the satisfaction that comes from eating delicious, nutritious meals that are made just for you!

Lemon Herb Grilled Chicken

For seniors trying to maintain a healthy and balanced diet, Grilled Lemon Herb Chicken is a tasty and protein-rich dish seasoned with fresh herbs and zesty lemon.

Value of Nutrition

- ✓ Approximately 150–200 kcal
- ✓ Approximately 25–30 grams of protein
- ✓ Fat: 5-8 grams, depending on the skin and cooking technique.
- ✓ Minimal, often less than a gram of carbohydrates
- ✓ Sodium: Depending on how much spice and marinade is used, the sodium concentration might change, although it often varies between 50 and 200 mg.

Ingredients:

- ✓ 4 skinless and boneless chicken breasts
- ✓ 2 tsp olive oil

- ✓ 2 minced garlic cloves
- ✓ One tablespoon of freshly chopped rosemary
- ✓ One tablespoon of freshly chopped thyme
- ✓ One lemon's juice and zest
- ✓ To taste, add salt and pepper.

Steps in Meal Preparation:

- ✓ To make a marinade, combine olive oil, chopped rosemary, thyme, zest, juice, salt, and pepper in a basin.
- ✓ Put the chicken breasts in a shallow dish or a plastic bag that can be sealed. Make sure the chicken is uniformly covered after pouring the marinade over it. Let it marinate for at least half an hour, or better still, all night.
- ✓ Grill at a medium-high temperature.
- ✓ Take the chicken out of the marinade and throw away any extra marinade. When the chicken Obtain an internal temperature of 165°F (74°C) and the juices flow clear, grill it for about 7–9 minutes on each side.

Jordan Marguire

✓ Before serving, let the chicken a few minutes to rest.

Why Seniors Benefit from It:

✓ **Protein Boost:** For muscle strength and repair, seniors frequently require higher protein intakes, and chicken offers a lean source.

✓ **Heart Health:** Grilled chicken, when prepared without added fats, supports heart health by being low in saturated fats.

✓ **Immune Support:** The vitamin C in lemons strengthens the immune system, which is important for the general health of elders.

✓ **Anti-inflammatory Properties:** Antioxidants included in fresh herbs may help lower inflammation, which is advantageous for elderly people.

Quinoa Salad with Mediterranean Flavors

A healthful and filling dinner choice for seniors, Mediterranean Quinoa Salad is a refreshing and nutrient-rich dish full of brilliant flavors from fresh veggies and tangy feta cheese.

Value of Nutrition

✓ Approximately 300 kcal of calories

✓ Protein: Approximately 10–12 grams

✓ Fat: 12–15 grams, primarily from feta cheese and olive oil, which are good sources of fat.

✓ About 35–40 grams of carbohydrates

✓ 6–8 grams of fiber help with digestion and increase feelings of fullness.

✓ More than half of the daily recommended consumption of vitamin C is provided, which supports immunological function.

✓ Calcium: Provides around 15–25% of the daily required amount and is good for bone health.

Jordan Marguire

Ingredients:

- ✓ One cup of washed quinoa
- ✓ 2 cups of veggie broth or water
- ✓ one chopped cucumber
- ✓ 1/2 a cup of cherry tomatoes
- ✓ ½ red onion, diced finely
- ✓ ½ cup of pitted and sliced Kalamata olives
- ✓ ½ cup of feta cheese in crumbles
- ✓ ¼ cup finely chopped fresh parsley
- ✓ ¼ cup finely chopped fresh mint leaves
- ✓ Three teaspoons of olive oil
- ✓ 2 tsp lemon juice
- ✓ To taste, add salt and pepper.

Steps in Meal Preparation:

- ✓ Give the quinoa a good rinse with cold water. Quinoa should be combined with water (or veggie broth) in a pot and heated to a boil. Once the quinoa is cooked and the water has been absorbed, reduce heat, cover, and simmer for 15 to 20 minutes. Give it time to cool.

✓ Cooked quinoa, diced cucumber, cherry tomatoes, red onion, chopped parsley, chopped mint, crumbled feta cheese, and Kalamata olives should all be combined in a big bowl.

✓ To make the dressing, combine the olive oil, lemon juice, salt, and pepper in a small bowl.

✓ Pour the dressing over the salad and gently toss to ensure that all of the items are coated.

✓ Serve right now or store in the fridge for later use.

Why Seniors Benefit from It:

✓ Nutrient-Dense: Packed with vital vitamins, minerals, and other nutrients that enhance seniors' general health.

✓ Digestive Health: A high fiber diet facilitates healthy digestion and gut flora.

✓ Bone Health: The calcium found in feta cheese is crucial for preserving bone density in older people.

✓ Low-Glycemic Index: Quinoa is better for seniors controlling their blood sugar levels since it has less of an effect on blood sugar levels.

Stir-fried veggies with tofu

Packed with a variety of veggies and plant-based protein, this colorful and nutrient-dense vegetable stir-fry with tofu is a tasty and filling lunch for seniors.

Value of Nutritionally

- ✓ Approximately 250–300 kcal of calories
- ✓ Protein: 15 to 20 grams
- ✓ Ten to twelve grams of fat, primarily from the beneficial fats in tofu and cooking oil.
- ✓ About 20 to 25 grams of carbohydrates
- ✓ 5-8 grams of fiber help with digestion and increase feelings of fullness.
- ✓ Rich in minerals such as calcium, iron, and potassium, as well as vitamins A, C, and K

Ingredients:

- ✓ 14 oz (400g) diced and drained firm tofu
- ✓ 2 cups of florets of broccoli
- ✓ One sliced red bell pepper

Jordan Marguire

✓ One sliced yellow bell pepper

✓ One cup of snap peas

✓ One sliced carrot

✓ three minced garlic cloves

✓ 2 teaspoons of soy sauce (if desired, low-sodium version)

✓ One tablespoon of sesame oil

✓ One tablespoon of olive oil

✓ One tablespoon cornstarch (to make the sauce thicker, optional)

✓ To taste, add salt and pepper.

Steps in Meal Preparation:

✓ Tofu should be pressed between paper towels to absorb extra moisture. Cube the food and set it aside.

✓ To make the sauce, combine the soy sauce, sesame oil, and cornstarch (if using) in a small bowl.

✓ In a large skillet or wok, heat the olive oil over medium-high heat. For 30 seconds, stir-fry the minced garlic.

- ✓ Cook the tofu cubes in the pan for 5 to 7 minutes, or until they are golden brown on both sides. Take out the tofu and place it aside in a skillet.
- ✓ Stir-fry broccoli, bell peppers, snap peas, and carrots in the same skillet for five to seven minutes, or until the veggies are crisp but still soft. Add a little more oil if necessary.
- ✓ Place the tofu back into the skillet and cover the tofu and veggies with the prepared sauce. In order to coat evenly and heat through, gently toss.
- ✓ To taste, add salt and pepper for seasoning.
- ✓ If preferred, serve the hot vegetable stir-fry with tofu over quinoa or brown rice.

Why Seniors Benefit from It:

- ✓ Plant-Based Protein: For seniors, tofu is a high-quality source of plant-based protein.
- ✓ Vegetables High in Nutrients: A variety of vegetables provide essential vitamins, minerals, and antioxidants for the well-being of the elderly.

- ✓ Low in Saturated Fat: Made with little to no oil, helping older people's hearts stay healthy.
- ✓ Digestive Health: Vegetables' high fiber content promotes a healthy digestive system.

Salad with Black Beans and Corn

This colorful, protein-rich Black Bean and Corn Salad gives seniors a tasty, filling supper alternative that is full of healthy components.

Value of Nutritionally:

- ✓ Approximately 200–250 kcal of calories
- ✓ Protein: Approximately 8–10 grams
- ✓ Approximately 5-7 grams of fat, largely from the good fats in olive oil.
- ✓ Approximately 30-35 grams of carbs
- ✓ 6–8 grams of fiber help with digestion and increase feelings of fullness.
- ✓ Rich in minerals including magnesium and potassium as well as vitamins A, C, and folate

Jordan Marguire

Ingredients:

- ✓ 2 cups of canned, drained, and rinsed black beans
- ✓ One cup of canned, frozen, or fresh sweet corn
- ✓ One sliced red bell pepper
- ✓ One chopped green bell pepper
- ✓ ½ red onion, diced finely
- ✓ ½ cup of freshly chopped cilantro
- ✓ 2 tsp olive oil
- ✓ Lime juice, 2 teaspoons
- ✓ One teaspoon of cumin powder
- ✓ To taste, add salt and pepper.
- ✓ Slices of avocado to serve, if desired

Steps in Meal Preparation:

- ✓ Add sweet corn, diced bell peppers, chopped red onion, chopped black beans, and fresh cilantro to a large mixing dish.
- ✓ To make the dressing, combine the olive oil, lime juice, ground cumin, salt, and pepper in a separate small bowl.

- ✓ Over the bean and vegetable combination, drizzle the dressing. Gently toss until all of the ingredients are uniformly covered.
- ✓ To enable the flavors to mingle, let the salad marinate in the fridge for at least half an hour.
- ✓ If preferred, top the cooled Black Bean and Corn Salad with sliced avocado.

Why Seniors Benefit from It:

- ✓ Plant-Based Protein: Black beans are an excellent source of plant-based protein that is appropriate for older citizens.
- ✓ Vegetables with color include fiber and antioxidants that are good for your general health.
- ✓ Heart-Healthy Fats: The addition of monounsaturated fats from olive oil is heart-healthy.
- ✓ Low-Glycemic Index: Vegetables and black beans provide slowly-releasing carbs that help seniors maintain their blood sugar.

Sweet Potato Fries in the Oven

Described as a delectable and nutrient-rich side dish for seniors, baked sweet potato fries are a healthier substitute for regular fries.

Value of Nutrition

- ✓ Approximately 150–200 kcal in calories
- ✓ Protein: Approximately 2-3 grams
- ✓ Fat: 4-6 grams, primarily in the form of good fats.
- ✓ Approximately 30-35 grams of carbs
- ✓ Fiber: Offers 4 to 6 grams, facilitating digestion and encouraging fullness.
- ✓ Minerals and vitamins: rich in potassium, vitamins A and C

Ingredients:

- ✓ Peel and chop two big sweet potatoes into fries.
- ✓ 2 tsp olive oil
- ✓ One tsp of paprika
- ✓ One-half teaspoon of powdered garlic

Jordan Marguire

- ✓ One-half teaspoon of onion powder
- ✓ To taste, add salt and pepper.

Steps in Meal Preparation:

- ✓ Adjust the oven temperature to 425°F (220°C) and place parchment paper on a baking pan.
- ✓ Sweet potato fries should be equally coated after being tossed in a big bowl of olive oil, paprika, onion powder, garlic powder, and salt.
- ✓ Arrange the seasoned sweet potato fries on the prepared baking sheet in a single layer, taking care not to pile them too high.
- ✓ Fries should be baked for 20 to 25 minutes in a preheated oven, turning them over halfway through, until they are crispy and golden brown.
- ✓ Before serving, take them out of the oven and allow them to cool somewhat.

Why Seniors Benefit from It:

✓ Nutrient-Rich Substitute: Sweet potatoes include antioxidants, vitamins, and minerals that are good for the health of older citizens.

✓ Fiber Content: Sweet potatoes have a high dietary fiber content that facilitates digestion and supports gut health.

✓ Less Saturated Fat: Baking reduces bad fats for seniors' heart health, as opposed to frying.

✓ Blood Sugar Regulation: Sweet potatoes help regulate blood sugar since they have a lower glycemic index.

✓ These tasty and nutritious baked sweet potato fries are a great substitute for conventional fries, giving seniors the critical nutrients they need without sacrificing flavor or enjoyment.

Greek Yogurt Parfait

The Greek Yogurt Parfait is a delightful and nutrient-rich breakfast or snack option filled with protein, probiotics, and fruits, offering seniors a delicious and healthful treat.

Nutritional Value of Nutrition

✓ Calories: Approximately 150-200 kcal

✓ Protein: Around 10-15 grams

✓ Fat: About 3-5 grams (mostly from yogurt and nuts)

✓ Carbohydrates: Roughly 20-25 grams

✓ Fiber: Provides 2-4 grams, depending on fruit and granola used

✓ Calcium: Rich in calcium, supporting bone health

Ingredients:

✓ 1 cup Greek yogurt (plain or flavored)

✓ ½ cup fresh berries (strawberries, blueberries, raspberries)

✓ ¼ cup granola

- ✓ 1 tablespoon honey or maple syrup (optional for added sweetness)
- ✓ 1 tablespoon chopped nuts (almonds, walnuts, or pecans)
- ✓ Fresh mint leaves for garnish (optional)

Meal Preparation Steps:

- ✓ In a glass or bowl, start by layering half of the Greek yogurt.
- ✓ Add a layer of fresh berries on top of the yogurt.
- ✓ Sprinkle a portion of granola over the berries.
- ✓ Drizzle honey or maple syrup (if using) for added sweetness.
- ✓ Add the remaining Greek yogurt as the next layer.
- ✓ Top with the rest of the berries, granola, and chopped nuts.
- ✓ Garnish with fresh mint leaves for a decorative touch.
- ✓ Serve the Greek Yogurt Parfait immediately as a breakfast option or refrigerate for a refreshing snack later.

Why It's Good for Seniors:

- ✓ Protein-Rich: Greek yogurt is a high-protein source vital for muscle strength and repair in seniors.
- ✓ Probiotics: Greek yogurt contains probiotics, promoting gut health and aiding digestion.
- ✓ Calcium Source: Beneficial for maintaining bone health, crucial for seniors' well-being.
- ✓ Antioxidants from Berries: Berries offer antioxidants that support overall health and may improve cognitive function.
- ✓ This Greek Yogurt Parfait offers a delicious and nutritious option for seniors, combining the goodness of yogurt, fruits, and nuts, making it an ideal breakfast or snack choice.

Garlic Herb Roasted Pork Tenderloin

Garlic Herb Roasted Pork Tenderloin is a flavorful and protein-packed dish seasoned with aromatic herbs and garlic, providing seniors with a hearty and satisfying meal option.

Value of Nutrition

- ✓ Calories: Approximately 200-250 kcal
- ✓ Protein: Around 25-30 grams
- ✓ Fat: About 8-10 grams (mostly from the pork loin)
- ✓ Carbohydrates: Minimal, around 2-3 grams
- ✓ Iron: Provides a significant portion of the daily recommended intake, supporting energy and vitality
- ✓ Vitamins: Contains B vitamins like B6 and B12 essential for overall health

Ingredients:

- ✓ 1 pork tenderloin (approximately 1 lb or 450g)
- ✓ 3 cloves garlic, minced
- ✓ 2 tablespoons olive oil
- ✓ 1 tablespoon fresh rosemary, chopped
- ✓ 1 tablespoon fresh thyme, chopped
- ✓ Salt and pepper to taste

Meal Preparation Steps:

- ✓ Preheat the oven to 400°F (200°C) and line a baking dish with foil.

- ✓ In a small bowl, mix minced garlic, olive oil, chopped rosemary, chopped thyme, salt, and pepper to create a marinade.
- ✓ Pat dry the pork tenderloin with paper towels. Place it in the prepared baking dish.
- ✓ Rub the marinade mixture all over the pork tenderloin, ensuring it's evenly coated.
- ✓ Roast in the preheated oven for 20-25 minutes or until the internal temperature reaches 145°F (63°C).
- ✓ Remove the pork from the oven and let it rest for 5-10 minutes before slicing.
- ✓ Slice the pork tenderloin into medallions and serve.

Why It's Good for Seniors:

- ✓ Protein Source: Pork tenderloin provides a lean source of protein vital for muscle health in seniors.
- ✓ Iron-Rich: Contains iron, essential for red blood cell production and energy levels.
- ✓ Herbs and Garlic: Aromatic herbs and garlic offer antioxidant and anti-inflammatory properties, beneficial for overall health.

✓ Ease of Digestion: Tender and lean pork cuts are easier to digest, suitable for aging digestive systems.

✓ This Garlic Herb Roasted Pork Tenderloin offers seniors a flavorful and nutrient-rich meal, providing essential proteins and nutrients for their overall health and vitality. Adjust seasoning and cooking time as needed based on preferences and desired doneness.

Ratatouille

Ratatouille is a delicious and colorful vegetable stew packed with nutrients and flavors, offering seniors a comforting and wholesome dish.

Value of Nutrition

✓ Calories: Approximately 150-200 kcal

✓ Protein: Around 3-5 grams

✓ Fat: About 8-10 grams (mostly from olive oil)

✓ Carbohydrates: Roughly 15-20 grams

✓ Fiber: Provides 5-8 grams, aiding digestion and promoting satiety

✓ Vitamins and Minerals: Rich in vitamins A, C, K, and potassium

Ingredients:

1 eggplant, diced

2 zucchinis, diced

1 bell pepper (red, yellow, or green), diced

1 onion, finely chopped

2 cloves garlic, minced

3 tomatoes, diced or 1 can (14 oz) diced tomatoes

2 tablespoons olive oil

1 teaspoon dried thyme

1 teaspoon dried basil

Salt and pepper to taste

Fresh basil leaves for garnish (optional)

Meal Preparation Steps:

✓ Heat olive oil in a large skillet or pot over medium heat.

- ✓ Add chopped onion and minced garlic. Sauté for 2-3 minutes until fragrant.
- ✓ Add diced eggplant, zucchini, and bell pepper to the skillet. Cook for 5-7 minutes until vegetables begin to soften.
- ✓ Stir in diced tomatoes (or canned tomatoes) along with dried thyme, dried basil, salt, and pepper.
- ✓ Cover the skillet and let the ratatouille simmer on low heat for 20-25 minutes, stirring occasionally, until vegetables are tender.
- ✓ Adjust seasoning if needed.
- ✓ Serve the Ratatouille hot, garnished with fresh basil leaves if desired.

Why It's Good for Seniors:

- ✓ Nutrient-Rich Vegetables: Eggplant, zucchini, bell peppers, and tomatoes offer vitamins, minerals, and antioxidants supporting senior health.
- ✓ Heart-Healthy Fats: Olive oil contributes healthy monounsaturated fats beneficial for heart health.

✓ Low-Calorie and High-Fiber: Provides a satisfying, low-calorie option with high fiber content, aiding in digestion and promoting fullness.

✓ Anti-Inflammatory Properties: Ingredients contain antioxidants that may help reduce inflammation, beneficial for aging individuals.

✓ This Ratatouille offers a flavorful and nutritious option for seniors, combining a variety of colorful vegetables and herbs, making it a comforting and healthful meal. Adjust seasoning and vegetables based on personal preferences.

Salmon with Dill Sauce

Rich in omega-3 fatty acids, salmon with dill sauce is a delectable and heart-healthy dish that provides seniors with a satisfying and nourishing alternative.

Value of Nutritionally:

✓ Approximately 250–300 kcal of calories

✓ 20–25 grams of protein

Jordan Marguire

- ✓ Fat: 15–20 grams, mostly from salmon, which is a good source of fat.
- ✓ Very little, fewer than 5 grams of carbohydrates
- ✓ Omega-3 Fatty Acids: High in omega-3s, which are good for the heart and brain
- ✓ A large amount of the daily required intake of vitamin D is provided by this nutrient, which is vital for healthy bones.

Ingredients:
- ✓ 4 fillets of salmon
- ✓ 2 tsp olive oil
- ✓ To taste, add salt and pepper.
- ✓ Greek yogurt, fresh dill, lemon juice, garlic, salt, and pepper are needed to make the dill sauce.

Steps in Meal Preparation:
- ✓ Adjust the oven temperature to 400°F (200°C) and place parchment paper on a baking pan.

✓ After putting the salmon fillets on the baking sheet that has been prepared, season with salt and pepper and drizzle with olive oil.

✓ Bake the salmon for 12 to 15 minutes, or until it is cooked through and flake readily with a fork, in an oven that has been warmed.

✓ While the salmon bakes, make the Dill Sauce in a bowl by combining Greek yogurt, minced garlic, lemon juice, chopped fresh dill, salt, and pepper.

✓ Top the cooked salmon with a generous amount of Dill Sauce and serve.

Why Seniors Benefit from It:

✓ Heart Health: The omega-3 fatty acids in salmon help to lower inflammation and support heart health.

✓ Bone Health: Offers vitamin D, which is essential for the calcium absorption and bone health of seniors.

✓ Provides a rich dose of both protein and healthy fats that are helpful for your general health.

Caramelized Veggie Soup

A warm and nutritious alternative for elders, Roasted Vegetable Soup is a pleasant and nutrient-rich dish full of various veggies.

Value of Nutritionally

- ✓ Approximately 150–200 kcal in calories
- ✓ Approximately 3-5 grams of protein
- ✓ Approximately 5-8 grams of fat, largely from olive oil
- ✓ About 20 to 25 grams of carbohydrates
- ✓ 5-8 grams of fiber help with digestion and increase feelings of fullness.
- ✓ Minerals and vitamins: Packed with antioxidants, minerals, and different kinds of vitamins

Ingredients:

- ✓ A variety of veggies (including bell peppers, tomatoes, onions, carrots, etc.)

Jordan Marguire

✓ Olive oil
✓ Cloves of garlic
✓ Broth made of vegetables
✓ Seasonings and herbs (pepper, salt, thyme, and rosemary)

Steps in Meal Preparation:
✓ Set oven temperature to 400°F, or 200°C.
✓ Slice a variety of veggies into small pieces and arrange them on a baking sheet.
✓ Add a drizzle of olive oil, minced garlic, salt, and pepper, along with herbs for seasoning.
✓ Bake the veggies for 25 to 30 minutes, or until they are soft and caramelized.
✓ Place the roasted veggies in a saucepan, cover with the vegetable broth, and heat through.
✓ Blend the soup with an immersion blender until it's smooth.
✓ Warm Roasted Vegetable Soup should be served.

Jordan Marguire

Why Seniors Benefit from It:
- ✓ Rich in nutrients: Packed with antioxidants, minerals, and vitamins to promote senior health.
- ✓ Fiber Content: A high fiber diet improves gut health and facilitates digestion.
- ✓ Low-Calorie Option: Offers elders a filling dinner that is low in calories.
- ✓ If you want me to go on to the next round of dishes from your list, please let me know!

Skewers of turkey with vegetables

Seniors may have a tasty and nutritious supper with these wonderful and protein-rich turkey and vegetable skewers that are packed with vibrant vegetables.

Value of Nutrition

- ✓ Approximately 200–250 kcal of calories
- ✓ 20–25 grams of protein
- ✓ 8 to 10 grams of fat, depending on how it's cooked.
- ✓ Approximately 10-15 grams of carbs

✓ Fiber: 3-5 grams, depending on the vegetables consumed

✓ Rich in potassium and a variety of other minerals as well as vitamins A, C, and K

Ingredients:

✓ Cubes of turkey or turkey breast

✓ Various veggies, including cherry tomatoes, bell peppers, onions, and zucchini

✓ Olive oil

✓ Herbs & spices (salt, pepper, paprika, oregano, and garlic powder)

✓ Wooden skewers should be soaked in water before grilling.

Steps in Meal Preparation:

✓ Turn the heat up to medium-high on the grill or grill pan.

✓ Cube the turkey and slice the veggies into skewer-friendly bits.

✓ Alternately thread veggies and turkey onto skewers.

- ✓ After giving the skewers a little olive oil brushing, add salt, pepper, herbs, and spices.
- ✓ Turning occasionally, grill the skewers for approximately 10 to 12 minutes, or until the turkey is cooked through and the veggies are soft.
- ✓ Warm up the skewers of turkey and vegetables.

Why Seniors Benefit from It:

- ✓ Lean Protein: Turkey provides a lean protein source that is essential for older muscle health.
- ✓ Assorted Vegetables: Offers antioxidants, vitamins, and minerals to enhance general health.
- ✓ Low-Fat Cooking Method: Grilling with little to no oil cuts down on extra fat, which is good for your heart.

Parmigiana di eggplant

With layers of eggplant, marinara sauce, and cheese, eggplant parmesan is a filling and gratifying dish that provides seniors with a tasty and cozy supper choice.

Value of Nutritionally

- ✓ Approximately 300–350 kcal of calories
- ✓ Protein: around 12–15 grams
- ✓ 15 to 20 grams of fat, largely from cheese and olive oil
- ✓ Approximately 30-35 grams of carbs
- ✓ Fiber: Depending on the size of the dish, provides 5-8 grams.
- ✓ Calcium: Cheese is a good source of calcium, which is good for bones.

Ingredients:

- ✓ Round slices of eggplant
- ✓ Almond meal can be used in place of breadcrumbs to make a low-carb version.

Jordan Marguire

- ✓ Eggs
- ✓ Sauce Marinara
- ✓ Cheese mozzarella
- ✓ Cheese Parmesan
- ✓ Olive oil
- ✓ Seasonings and herbs (garlic powder, oregano, basil, salt, and pepper)

Steps in Meal Preparation:

- ✓ Turn the oven on to 375°F, or 190°C.
- ✓ Coat the eggplant pieces with almond flour or breadcrumbs after dipping them into beaten eggs.
- ✓ Slices of eggplant should be pan-fried in hot olive oil until they get golden brown on both sides.
- ✓ Arrange eggplant slices, marinara sauce, mozzarella, Parmesan, and herbs in a baking dish. Continue layering until all the ingredients are utilized, and then top with cheese.
- ✓ Bake for 25 to 30 minutes, or until the cheese is bubbling and brown.
- ✓ Warm up the eggplant parmesan.

Why Seniors Benefit from It:

- ✓ Benefits of Eggplant: Provides fiber and antioxidants that support heart health and digestion.
- ✓ Cheese High in Calcium: Gives seniors the calcium they need to maintain healthy bones.
- ✓ Vegetarian Option: Ideal for older citizens seeking high-protein, vegetarian meals.

Chicken Breast Stuffed with Feta and Spinach

Seniors may have a tasty and nourishing lunch with this dish of spinach and feta stuffed chicken breast, which is aromatic and high in protein.

Value of Nutrition

- ✓ Approximately 250–300 kcal of calories
- ✓ About 25–30 grams of protein
- ✓ 10 to 15 grams of fat, largely from cheese and chicken.

Jordan Marguire

- ✓ Carbohydrates: Very little, three to five grams
- ✓ Provides some of the daily required intake of both calcium and iron, which is good for energy and bone health.

Ingredients:
- ✓ Breasts of chicken
- ✓ fresh leaves of spinach
- ✓ Feta cheese
- ✓ Powdered garlic
- ✓ Olive oil
- ✓ To taste, add salt and pepper.

Steps in Meal Preparation:
- ✓ Turn the oven on to 375°F, or 190°C.
- ✓ Gently slice the chicken breasts in half lengthwise, taking care not to cut all the way through.
- ✓ Add salt, pepper, and garlic powder into the chicken breasts to season the insides.

- ✓ Place a few handfuls of fresh spinach leaves and some crumbled feta cheese inside each chicken breast.
- ✓ If necessary, fasten the chicken breasts closed with toothpicks.
- ✓ In a pan that is ovensafe, warm the olive oil over medium-high heat.
- ✓ Sear the filled chicken breasts until browned, about two to three minutes per side.
- ✓ Place the pan in the oven that has been warmed, and bake for 20 to 25 minutes, or until the chicken is well done.

Why Seniors Benefit from It:
- ✓ Source of Protein: Lean protein, like as chicken, is essential for the health of elderly muscles.
- ✓ Calcium and Leafy Greens: Iron and calcium found in spinach are good for healthy bones and general vigor.

✓ Nutrient-Rich and Flavorful: Feta cheese contributes vital nutrients to the meal while also giving it taste and richness.

Zucchini Noodles with Pesto

Seniors now have a low-carb, high-nutrient dinner alternative with zucchini noodles with pesto, a light and refreshing take on classic pasta.

Value of Nutritionally

✓ Approximately 150–200 kcal in calories

✓ Approximately 3-5 grams of protein

✓ 10–12 grams of fat, largely from almonds and olive oil

✓ Approximately 10-15 grams of carbs

✓ Fiber: Depending on the size of the meal, provides 2-4 grams.

✓ Minerals and vitamins: Packed with potassium and vitamins A, C, and K

Jordan Marguire

Ingredients:

- ✓ spiralized zucchini to make noodles
- ✓ (Homemade or store-bought) pesto sauce
- ✓ Walnuts or pine nuts (as garnish)
- ✓ fresh sprigs of basil (to garnish)

Steps in Meal Preparation:

- ✓ Using a spiralizer or julienne peeler, spiralize zucchini into noodles.
- ✓ When the pan is hot, add the zucchini noodles.
- ✓ The zucchini noodles should be sautéed for two to three minutes, or until they are slightly crunchy but still soft.
- ✓ After turning off the heat, remove the pan and toss the zucchini noodles in the pesto sauce until well covered.
- ✓ Present Pesto-topped zucchini noodles with walnuts or pine nuts and fresh basil leaves as garnish.

Why Seniors Benefit from It:

✓ Low-Carb Option: Zucchini is a low-carb substitute for regular spaghetti.

✓ Nutrient-Dense: Light and simple to digest, zucchini is a good source of vitamins and minerals.

✓ Healthy Fats in Pesto: Nuts and olive oil combine to create a pesto that is rich in heart-healthy fats.

Salad of tuna and white beans

A tasty and well-balanced dinner for seniors, tuna and white bean salad is full of healthy components and high in protein.

Value of Nutrition

✓ Approximately 200–250 kcal of calories

✓ Protein: 15 to 20 grams

✓ Approximately 5-8 grams of fat, largely from olive oil and tuna.

✓ About 20 to 25 grams of carbohydrates

Jordan Marguire

- ✓ 6–8 grams of fiber help with digestion and increase feelings of fullness.
- ✓ Minerals and vitamins: Vegetables and beans are a great source of many minerals and vitamins.

Ingredients:

- ✓ Tuna canned
- ✓ Rinse and drain white beans (cannellini or navy beans).
- ✓ Half a cherry tomato
- ✓ Slices of red onion, thinly
- ✓ Halved and pitted Kalamata olives
- ✓ Olive oil
- ✓ Juice from lemons
- ✓ chopped fresh parsley
- ✓ To taste, add salt and pepper.

Steps in Meal Preparation:

- ✓ Drained canned tuna, white beans, cherry tomatoes, chopped red onion, and halved Kalamata olives should all be combined in a big mixing dish.

- ✓ Pour lemon juice and olive oil on top of the mixture.
- ✓ Add the salt, pepper, and freshly chopped parsley.
- ✓ Gently toss until all items are thoroughly mixed.
- ✓ The Tuna and White Bean Salad should be served cold.

Why Seniors Benefit from It:

- ✓ Rich in Protein: White beans and tuna provide a significant amount of protein that is essential for the health of elderly muscles.
- ✓ High Fiber Content: The fiber in beans and vegetables helps with digestion and supports gut health.
- ✓ Omega-3 Fatty Acids: Heart and brain health-promoting omega-3s may be found in tuna.

Fish Baked with Herbs

Seniors have a tasty and nutritious dinner choice with Baked Cod with Herbs, a light and delectable fish dish seasoned with herbs.

Value of Nutrition

- ✓ Approximately 150–200 kcal in calories
- ✓ 20–25 grams of protein
- ✓ Fat: 5-8 grams, primarily from the fish's healthful fats.
- ✓ Carbohydrates: Very little, perhaps 2-3 grams
- ✓ Rich in omega-3 fatty acids, which are good for heart health

Ingredients:

- ✓ Fillets of cod
- ✓ Olive oil
- ✓ Fresh herbs, such thyme, dill, or parsley
- ✓ Juice from lemons
- ✓ minced cloves of garlic

✓ To taste, add salt and pepper.

Steps in Meal Preparation:

✓ Turn the oven on to 375°F, or 190°C.

✓ Cod fillets should be patted dry with paper towels before being put on a baking dish covered with parchment paper.

✓ Over the cod fillets, drizzle some olive oil and lemon juice.

✓ On top, equally distribute the minced garlic, chopped fresh herbs, salt, and pepper.

✓ Bake the fish for 12 to 15 minutes in a preheated oven, or until it is cooked through and flake easily with a fork.

✓ Warm Baked Cod with Herbs should be served.

Why Seniors Benefit from It:

✓ High-quality Protein: Cod is a lean protein source that is essential for elderly citizens' muscles to remain healthy.

- ✓ Rich in omega-3 fatty acids, which may help lower inflammation and promote heart health.
- ✓ Light and Simple to Digest: Cod is a mild fish that is good for elderly people's digestive systems.
- ✓ These recipes provide seniors with a range of tasty, nourishing, and simple-to-make meals.

Pilaf of brown rice with vegetables

Seniors may have a satisfying and tasty dinner with Brown Rice Pilaf with veggies, a rich and healthy recipe that combines whole grains and vibrant veggies.

Value of Nutrition

- ✓ Approximately 200–250 kcal of calories
- ✓ Approximately 5-8 grams of protein
- ✓ Fat: 5-7 grams, primarily in the form of good fats or olive oil.
- ✓ Approximately 30-35 grams of carbs
- ✓ Fiber: Offers four to six grams, facilitating digestion and encouraging fullness.

Jordan Marguire

✓ Minerals and vitamins: Rich in a variety of minerals and vitamins from whole grains and veggies.

Ingredients:

✓ Grains of brown rice
✓ A variety of veggies, such as bell peppers, carrots, and peas
✓ Finely sliced onion
✓ Minced garlic
✓ Olive oil
✓ Broth made from vegetables or chicken
✓ Seasonings and herbs (parsley, thyme, salt, and pepper)

Steps in Meal Preparation:

✓ After rinsing with cold water, set aside the brown rice.
✓ Add the minced garlic and continue to sauté for an additional minute after adding the chopped onions to a pan of heated olive oil over medium heat.

- ✓ Stir the brown rice in the pan to evenly distribute the oil over the grains.
- ✓ Add the vegetable or chicken broth, making sure the rice-to-liquid ratio is as directed on the box.
- ✓ Add the herbs, salt, pepper, and variety of veggies.
- ✓ Once the rice is soft and the liquid has been absorbed, cover the pan and simmer.
- ✓ Serve the brown rice pilaf with vegetables hot after fluffing the rice with a fork.

Why Seniors Benefit from It:

- ✓ Benefits of Whole Grains: Brown rice gives you the fiber and nutrition your digestive system needs.
- ✓ Vegetable Nutrients: A variety of vegetables provide antioxidants, vitamins, and minerals that promote elder health.
- ✓ Heart-Healthy Option: Seniors' heart health is enhanced by consuming healthy grains and veggies.

Pizza with Cauliflower Crust

Seniors now have a tasty and healthy option in cauliflower crust pizza, which is low in carbohydrates and gluten.

Value of Nutrition

- ✓ About 200–250 calories (depending on the toppings).
- ✓ Protein: Approximately 8–10 grams
- ✓ 10–12 grams of fat (varies depending on cheese and toppings)
- ✓ About 10 to 15 grams of carbohydrates, depending on the toppings and sauce.
- ✓ Fiber: Depending on the crust and toppings, provides three to five grams.
- ✓ Minerals and vitamins: Provides a variety of minerals from the toppings and vitamins from the cauliflower.

Ingredients:

- ✓ Grated cauliflower

- ✓ Whites or eggs?
- ✓ Cheese (parmesan, mozzarella)
- ✓ Low-sugar or homemade pizza sauce
- ✓ Add-ons for pizza, such as veggies and lean meats.
- ✓ Seasonings and herbs (garlic powder, basil, and oregano)

Steps in Meal Preparation:

- ✓ Adjust the oven temperature to 425°F (220°C) and place parchment paper on a baking pan.
- ✓ Using a food processor or grater, shred the cauliflower.
- ✓ Grated cauliflower should be steamed or microwaved, let to cool, and then any extra moisture should be squeezed out using a fresh kitchen towel.
- ✓ To make a dough, combine the cauliflower, cheese, eggs, or egg whites, and herbs in a bowl.
- ✓ To make the pizza crust, press the dough onto the baking sheet that has been prepared.
- ✓ For 15 to 20 minutes, or until it is firm and golden, bake the cauliflower crust in a preheated oven.

✓ After removing the crust, add the pizza sauce, cheese, and toppings. Bake it again until the cheese has melted and the toppings are cooked.

Why Seniors Benefit from It:
✓ Low-Carb Option: For seniors limiting their carbohydrate consumption, cauliflower crust provides a lower-carb option to classic pizza.

✓ Vegetable-Based: Contains cauliflower, which contributes fiber, vitamins, and minerals.

✓ Tasty and customizable: Seniors may eat pizza and keep an eye on the ingredients for a more healthful dinner.

Curry with Lentil and Vegetables

Seniors may have a satisfying and fragrant supper with this savory and filling lentil and vegetable curry, which is loaded with protein and a variety of veggies.

Value of Nutrition:

✓ Approximately 250–300 kcal of calories

✓ Protein: around 12–15 grams

✓ 8–10 grams of fat, usually from oil or coconut milk.

✓ Approximately 30-35 grams of carbs

✓ Eight to ten grams of fiber help with digestion and increase feelings of fullness.

✓ Minerals and vitamins: Vegetables and lentils are a great source of several vitamins and minerals.

Ingredients:

✓ Red or green lentils

✓ a variety of veggies, such as spinach, carrots, and bell peppers

✓ finely sliced onion

✓ minced garlic

✓ Curry paste or powder

✓ Milk from coconuts

✓ Olive oil

✓ To taste, add salt and pepper.

Steps in Meal Preparation:

- ✓ Cook lentils as directed on the box until they are soft, then drain and put aside.

- ✓ In a skillet set over medium heat, sauté chopped onions in olive oil until they become translucent. Next, add minced garlic and continue cooking for an additional minute.

- ✓ When the veggies start to soften, add the assortment and simmer.

- ✓ Add curry paste or powder and stir until the veggies are equally coated.

- ✓ After adding the cooked lentils and coconut milk, mix everything together.

- ✓ Simmer the curry for several minutes to allow the spices to combine and the sauce to get thicker.

- ✓ Serve the hot lentil and vegetable curry hot over rice or over naan bread after adjusting the flavor with salt and pepper.

Jordan Marguire

Why Seniors Benefit from It:

✓ Rich in Protein: Lentils offer a plant-based source of protein that is vital for the health of muscles.

✓ Variety of veggies: A variety of veggies include antioxidants, vitamins, and minerals to enhance senior health.

✓ Rich in Nutrients and Fiber: Vegetables and lentils offer fiber that improves general health and aids with digestion.

Bell Peppers Stuffed

Stuffed bell peppers provide seniors with a good and filling lunch. They are colorful and nutritious, packed with a savory combination of rice, protein, and veggies.

Value of Nutrition

✓ Approximately 250–300 kcal of calories

✓ About 10–15 grams of protein

✓ 8 to 10 grams of fat, depending on the cheese and filling.

Jordan Marguire

- ✓ Approximately 30-35 grams of carbs
- ✓ 4-6 grams of fiber, depending on the filling
- ✓ Minerals and vitamins: Packed with different nutrients from filling

Ingredients

- ✓ Bell peppers (many hues)
- ✓ Ground meat (vegetable protein for vegetarians, or beef, turkey, or both)
- ✓ Cooked quinoa or rice
- ✓ Diced onion
- ✓ minced garlic
- ✓ Diced tomatoes or tomato sauce
- ✓ Cheese (topping optional)
- ✓ Seasonings and herbs (paprika, oregano, basil, salt, and pepper)

Steps in Meal Preparation:

- ✓ Adjust the oven temperature to 375°F (190°C) and get a baking dish ready.

- ✓ Cut off the bell peppers' tops, then remove the seeds and membranes.
- ✓ Cook minced garlic and chopped onions with ground beef in a pan until the meat is browned.
- ✓ Toss thoroughly to combine cooked rice or quinoa, diced tomatoes or tomato sauce, herbs, and spices in the pan.
- ✓ The meat and rice mixture should be poured into each bell pepper until it reaches the top.
- ✓ Fill the bell peppers with stuffing and cover the dish with foil.
- ✓ After baking for 25 to 30 minutes, take off the foil, top with cheese, if using, and continue baking for another 5 to 10 minutes, or until the cheese is melted and the peppers are soft.

Why Seniors Benefit from It:
- ✓ Bell peppers are a colorful and nutrient-dense food that are good for senior health since they include vitamins and antioxidants.

✓ Protein and Whole Grain: Rice or quinoa provides vital nutrients, while animal or plant-based protein fills the gap.

✓ Versatile and Filling: Easily altered to fit certain dietary requirements with a variety of fillings.

Mango Salsa Chicken

Mango Salsa Chicken is a tasty and colorful recipe that combines the savory grilled chicken with the sweetness of mango, providing seniors with a satisfying and nourishing meal.

Value of Nutrition:

✓ Approximately 250–300 kcal of calories

✓ About 25–30 grams of protein

✓ 8 to 10 grams of fat, depending on how it's cooked.

✓ About 20 to 25 grams of carbohydrates

✓ Fiber: Depending on the size of the meal, provides 2-4 grams.

✓ Minerals and vitamins: Mango and veggies are a good source of vitamin C and other minerals.

Ingredients:
- ✓ Thighs or breasts of chicken
- ✓ Diced ripe mango
- ✓ Chopped red bell pepper
- ✓ finely sliced red onion
- ✓ chopped fresh cilantro
- ✓ Lime juice
- ✓ Olive oil
- ✓ To taste, add salt and pepper.

Steps in Meal Preparation:
- ✓ Turn the heat up to medium-high on the grill or grill pan.
- ✓ After adding salt, pepper, and olive oil to the chicken, grill it for 6 to 8 minutes on each side, or until it is cooked through.

Jordan Marguire

- ✓ Diced mango, bell pepper, sliced red onion, chopped cilantro, lime juice, and a dash of salt should all be combined in a dish.
- ✓ To make the mango salsa, thoroughly mix.
- ✓ Before serving, spread some mango salsa over the cooked chicken.

Why Seniors Benefit from It:

- ✓ Lean Protein Source: One important lean protein source for the health of muscles is grilled chicken.
- ✓ Mangos are rich in vitamin C, which supports the immune system and general health.
- ✓ Fresh and Flavorful: The taste of mango salsa combined with chicken is delightfully light and delicious

Broccoli and Cheddar Frittata

Cheddar and Broccoli Seniors have a delicious and high-protein dinner choice in frittata, a tasty and simple dish made with cheese and veggies.

Value of Nutritional

- ✓ Approximately 200–250 kcal of calories
- ✓ Protein: 15 to 20 grams
- ✓ 10–12 grams of fat, largely from cheese and eggs.
- ✓ About 5-8 grams of carbohydrates
- ✓ Fiber: Depending on the size of the meal, provides 2-4 grams.
- ✓ Rich in minerals and vitamins A, K, and other nutrients from eggs and broccoli

Ingredient:

- ✓ Eggs
- ✓ florets of broccoli
- ✓ grated cheddar cheese
- ✓ finely sliced onion

Jordan Marguire

- ✓ (Optional) milk
- ✓ Butter or olive oil
- ✓ Seasonings and herbs (pepper, salt, thyme, and parsley)

Steps in Meal Preparation:

- ✓ Set the oven's temperature to 175°C/350°F.
- ✓ Chop the onion and sauté the broccoli florets in an ovenproof pan until they become slightly soft
- ✓ Beat eggs with shredded cheddar cheese, herbs, and milk (if using) in a bowl.
- ✓ Over the onions and broccoli that have been sautéed in the skillet, pour the egg mixture.
- ✓ Cook for a few minutes on the stovetop, or until the edges begin to solidify.
- ✓ Place the pan in the oven that has been prepared, and bake for 15 to 20 minutes, or until the frittata is set and has a hint of color on top.

Why Seniors Benefit from It:

- ✓ Rich in Protein: Cheese and eggs provide the protein needed to maintain healthy muscles.
- ✓ Vegetable Enriched: Broccoli provides antioxidants, fiber, and vitamins that are good for your general health.
- ✓ Flexible and Simple to Make: Frittatas may be easily customized to incorporate desired tastes and veggies.

Sweet Potato Fries in the Oven

Seniors now have a tasty and wholesome side dish or snack choice in baked sweet potato fries, which are a healthier substitute for conventional fries.

Value of Nutrition:

- ✓ Approximately 150–200 kcal in calories
- ✓ Protein: Approximately two to three grams
- ✓ 3-5 grams of fat, depending on serving size
- ✓ Approximately 30-35 grams of carbs

✓ Depending on serving size, 4-6 grams of fiber are provided.

✓ Vitamins and Minerals: Sweet potatoes are a rich source of potassium, vitamin A, and other minerals.

Ingredient:

✓ Cut sweet potatoes into the shape of fries.

✓ Olive oil

✓ Paprika

✓ Powdered garlic

✓ To taste, add salt and pepper.

Steps in Meal Preparation:

✓ Adjust the oven temperature to 425°F (220°C) and place parchment paper on a baking pan.

✓ In a mixing dish, toss the sweet potato fries with the olive oil, paprika, garlic powder, salt, and pepper until well coated.

✓ Arrange the spiced sweet potato fries in a single layer on the baking sheet that has been preheated.

- ✓ Fries should be baked for 20 to 25 minutes in a preheated oven, rotating them halfway through, or until they are crispy and golden brown.
- ✓ Hot baked sweet potato fries are a great snack or side dish.

Why Seniors Benefit from It:

- ✓ Rich in Nutrients: Sweet potatoes are a good source of antioxidants, vitamins, and minerals for senior health.
- ✓ Lower in Fat: Baking preserves taste and texture while cutting back on needless fat intake compared to frying.
- ✓ Fiber Content: Provides fiber to support gut health and help in digestion.

Grilled Chicken with Greek Salad

Greek salad with grilled chicken is a nutrient-dense, hydrating dish that makes a light and filling dinner for seniors. It is laden with fresh vegetables and grilled chicken.

Value of Nutrition:
- ✓ Approximately 250–300 kcal of calories
- ✓ About 25–30 grams of protein
- ✓ 8–10 grams of fat, primarily from chicken and olive oil
- ✓ Approximately 15-20 grams of carbs
- ✓ Depending on serving size, 4-6 grams of fiber are provided.
- ✓ Rich in minerals and vitamins A, C, and K, as well as other nutrients from chicken and veggies

Ingredients:
- ✓ Sliced, grilled chicken breast
- ✓ Diced cucumbers
- ✓ Diced tomatoes
- ✓ Slices of red onion, thinly
- ✓ Olives kalamata
- ✓ Feta cheese, broken up

- ✓ Olive oil
- ✓ Vinegar of red wine
- ✓ Either dried or fresh oregano
- ✓ To taste, add salt and pepper.

Steps in Meal Preparation:

- ✓ Diced cucumbers, tomatoes, red onion slices cut thinly, crumbled feta cheese, and Kalamata olives should all be combined in a big bowl.
- ✓ Add pieces of grilled chicken to the salad.
- ✓ After drizzling the salad with red wine vinegar and olive oil, add salt, pepper, and either dried or fresh oregano.
- ✓ Gently toss the ingredients until thoroughly mixed.
- ✓ Present the chilled Greek Salad beside the Grilled Chicken.

Why Seniors Benefit from It:

- ✓ Protein Source: Lean protein from grilled chicken is essential for the health of muscles.

- ✓ Vegetable Enriched: Antioxidants, vitamins, and minerals that are good for your general health may be found in fresh veggies.
- ✓ Light and Refreshing: A filling yet light salad choice that may accommodate different dietary requirements.

Curry with Chickpeas and Spinach

Seniors may have a filling and substantial supper with this tasty and healthful vegetarian dish of chickpea and spinach curry, which is loaded with protein, fiber, and vital elements.

Value of Nutrition (per serving):

- ✓ Approximately 250–300 kcal of calories
- ✓ About 10–15 grams of protein
- ✓ 8–10 grams of fat, usually from oil or coconut milk.
- ✓ Approximately 30-35 grams of carbs
- ✓ Eight to ten grams of fiber help with digestion and increase feelings of fullness.

Jordan Marguire

✓ Minerals and vitamins: Chickpeas and spinach are a great source of several minerals and vitamins.

Ingredients:

✓ Cooked or canned chickpeas

✓ Fresh leaves of spinach

✓ Finely sliced onion

✓ Minced garlic

✓ Diced tomatoes or tomato paste

✓ Milk from coconuts

✓ Olive oil

✓ Curry paste or powder

✓ Herbs & spices (salt, pepper, turmeric, coriander, and cumin)

Steps in Meal Preparation:

✓ In a skillet set over medium heat, sauté chopped onions in olive oil until they become translucent. Next, add minced garlic and continue cooking for an additional minute.

✓ For a minute, roast the spices in the pan by adding the curry powder or paste.

✓ Add the chopped tomatoes or tomato paste, then the coconut milk, and boil.

✓ After adding the chickpeas, let the mixture a few minutes to simmer.

✓ Cook the fresh spinach leaves in the curry until they wilt.

✓ Add more salt, pepper, and any desired spices to adjust the seasoning.

✓ Serve heated naan bread or rice alongside the chickpea and spinach curry.

Why Seniors Benefit from It:

✓ Plant-Based Protein: An essential source of plant-based protein for the health of muscles is chickpeas.

✓ Iron-Rich Spinach: Among its many health and energy-promoting components, spinach also contains iron.

✓ Fiber and Nutrients: Rich in fiber, spinach and chickpeas support healthy digestion and general well-being.

Portobello Mushrooms Stuffed

Seniors have a filling and adaptable dinner choice with stuffed portobello mushrooms, a tasty and healthy dish packed with a savory combination.

Value of Nutrition:

✓ Approximately 150–200 kcal in calories

✓ Protein: Approximately 8–10 grams

✓ Fat: 5-7 grams, depending on the components of the filling.

✓ Approximately 10-15 grams of carbs

✓ Fiber: 2-4 grams, depending on the components of the filling

✓ Minerals and vitamins: Packed with a variety of minerals from the filling materials and mushrooms

Jordan Marguire

Ingredient:
✓ Portobello fungi
✓ Ingredients for stuffing (quinoa, veggies, cheese, herbs, etc.)
✓ Butter or olive oil
✓ Herbs and spices (salt, pepper, thyme, onion, and garlic powder)

Steps in Meal Preparation:
✓ Warm up the oven to 375°F, or 190°C, and get a baking sheet ready.
✓ Clean the caps of Portobello mushrooms and remove the stems.
✓ To make a filling, combine stuffing components (cooked quinoa, sautéed veggies, cheese, herbs, etc.) in a dish.
✓ Apply a thin layer of melted butter or olive oil to the mushroom tops.
✓ Stuff the stuffing mixture into each mushroom cap.
✓ After placing the filled mushrooms on the baking sheet, bake them in the preheated oven for 15 to 20

minutes, or until the filling is well cooked and the mushrooms are soft.

Why Seniors Benefit from It:

✓ Low-Calorie Option: For seniors managing their calorie intake, portobello mushrooms provide a low-calorie stuffing basis.

✓ Flexible and High in Nutrients: The filling may be tailored with a range of nutritious ingredients to meet dietary requirements and personal tastes.

✓ Delicious and Simple to Make: Stuffed Portobello Mushrooms are a simple and tasty dinner option.

Stir-fried Sesame Ginger Tofu

Sesame Ginger Tofu Stir-Fry is a tasty, high-protein dish that is packed with veggies, making it a healthy and delectable supper option for seniors.

Value of Nutrition:

✓ Approximately 250–300 kcal of calories

- ✓ Protein: 15 to 20 grams
- ✓ 10–12 grams of fat, largely from tofu and sesame oil
- ✓ About 20 to 25 grams of carbohydrates
- ✓ Depending on serving size, 4-6 grams of fiber are provided.
- ✓ Minerals and vitamins: Packed with a variety of nutrients from veggies and tofu

Ingredients:
- ✓ Cubed, firm tofu
- ✓ A variety of veggies (carrots, broccoli, bell peppers, etc.)
- ✓ Sliced onion
- ✓ Minced garlic
- ✓ Ginger, finely chopped
- ✓ Tamari or soy sauce
- ✓ Oil from sesame
- ✓ Vinegar made from rice
- ✓ Cornstarch, if desired, to thicken
- ✓ Sunflower seeds (as a garnish)
- ✓ Green onions (as a garnish)

Jordan Marguire

Steps in Meal Preparation:

- ✓ Cut tofu into cubes after pressing to eliminate extra moisture.
- ✓ In a skillet or wok, warm the sesame oil over medium-high heat.
- ✓ Grated ginger and chopped garlic should be sautéed until aromatic.
- ✓ Stir-fry the cubed tofu and chopped onion until the tofu begins to take on light brown hues.
- ✓ Stir-fry the mixed veggies in the pan until they become crisp and tender.
- ✓ Combine rice vinegar, cornstarch, and soy sauce or tamari in a small basin.
- ✓ Once the sauce has thickened and covered the ingredients, pour the sauce mixture into the pan and stir continuously.
- ✓ Before serving, garnish with sliced green onions and sesame seeds.

Jordan Marguire

Why Seniors Benefit from It:

✓ Protein-Packed Tofu: Tofu is a vital plant-based source of protein for healthy muscles.

✓ Variety of veggies: A variety of veggies include antioxidants, vitamins, and minerals that promote elder health.

✓ Rich in Nutrients and Low in Calories: A tasty dish that is high in nutrients yet low in calorie

Cucumber Avocado Soup

Cucumber Avocado Soup is a light and hydrating dinner choice for seniors. It is a pleasant, creamy chilled soup full of nutritional ingredients.

Value of Nutrition:

✓ Approximately 150–200 kcal in calories

✓ Protein: Approximately two to three grams

✓ 10–12 grams of fat, largely from avocado and olive oil

- ✓ Approximately 10-15 grams of carbsDepending on serving size, 4-6 grams of fiber are provided.
- ✓ Rich in vitamins K and C as well as other minerals from avocado and cucumber

Ingredients

- ✓ Sliced and peeled cucumbers
- ✓ Diced and peeled ripe avocados
- ✓ Greek or coconut yogurt (for a plant-based substitute)
- ✓ freshly squeezed lemon juice
- ✓ Olive oil
- ✓ For garnish, use fresh cilantro or dill.
- ✓ To taste, add salt and pepper.

Steps in Meal Preparation:

- ✓ Greek yogurt, diced avocados, sliced cucumbers, fresh lemon juice, olive oil, salt, and pepper should all be combined in a blender.
- ✓ Mix the ingredients until they are creamy and smooth.

- ✓ Taste and adjust with extra salt, pepper, or lemon juice, if needed.
- ✓ Chill the Cucumber Avocado Soup in the refrigerator.
- ✓ Garnish the soup with cilantro or fresh dill.

Why Seniors Benefit from It:
- ✓ Rich in nutrients and hydrating: Avocados and cucumbers provide vital nutrients and hydration.
- ✓ Healthy Fats from Avocados: Avocados are a good source of heart-healthy fats.
- ✓ Light and Easy to Digest: During the warmer months, seniors can benefit from this smooth and pleasant soup.

Turkey Meatballs Baked

Seniors have a flexible and filling dinner choice with baked turkey meatballs, a lean and tasty protein source.

Value of Nutrition

Jordan Marguire

- ✓ Approximately 200–250 kcal of calories
- ✓ Protein: 15 to 20 grams
- ✓ 8–10 grams of fat, depending on how lean the ground turkey is
- ✓ About 5-8 grams of carbohydrates
- ✓ Depending on serving size, 1-3 grams of fiber are provided.
- ✓ Minerals and vitamins: Provides a range of nutrients from lean turkey ground and spices.

Ingredients:

- ✓ Turkey that is lean
- ✓ A grain of bread or oat flour
- ✓ finely sliced onion
- ✓ minced garlic
- ✓ Egg
- ✓ Cheese Parmesan (optional)
- ✓ Herbs (parsley, basil, oregano, salt, and pepper) and spices

Jordan Marguire

Steps in Meal Preparation:

✓ Adjust the oven temperature to 400°F (200°C) and place parchment paper on a baking pan.

✓ Lean ground turkey, oat flour or breadcrumbs, minced onion, chopped garlic, beaten egg, grated Parmesan cheese (if used), and herbs should all be combined in a bowl.

✓ Don't overmix; just stir until everything is fully blended.

✓ Form the mixture into meatballs and transfer to the baking sheet that has been preheated.

✓ Bake the meatballs for 15 to 20 minutes, or until they are cooked through and have a light brown color, in a preheated oven.

Why Seniors Benefit from It:

✓ Lean Protein Source: One important source of protein for the health of muscles is lean ground turkey.

- ✓ Low in Fat: Ideal for senior dietary needs, lean turkey meatballs deliver protein without being too fattening.
- ✓ Versatile and Simple to Make: You may serve baked turkey meatballs with a variety of sauces or incorporate them into salads, sandwiches, and pasta dishes.

Avocado Salad

Ripe tomatoes, creamy mozzarella, aromatic basil, and a balsamic sauce come together to create a fresh and colorful caprese salad.

Value of Nutrition

- ✓ 180 kcal of calories
- ✓ 10 g of protein
- ✓ Five grams of carbohydrates
- ✓ 12 grams of fat
- ✓ 2 g of fiber

- ✓ Ingredient:
- ✓ fresh tomatoes
- ✓ recent mozzarella cheese
- ✓ fresh leaves of basil
- ✓ Balsamic reduction or glaze
- ✓ Olive oil
- ✓ To taste, add salt and pepper.

Steps in Meal Preparation:
- ✓ Cut fresh mozzarella and tomatoes into slices of the same size.
- ✓ Place slices of mozzarella, tomato, and fresh basil on a platter.
- ✓ Drizzle with balsamic glaze and olive oil.
- ✓ Before serving, add some salt and pepper to taste.

Why Seniors Can Benefit from It:
- ✓ Rich in nutrients: Tomatoes contain antioxidants, while mozzarella provides calcium and protein, which helps older people's bones stay strong.

- ✓ Low-Calorie Option: For seniors managing their calorie consumption, a low-calorie dish that nevertheless offers vital nutrients and tastes is appropriate.
- ✓ simple to Chew: Seniors will find this salad simple to chew and digest due to the soft texture of the mozzarella and tomatoes.

Berries on Whole Grain Pancakes

Made with whole grain flour and topped with a mix of fresh berries, Whole Grain Pancakes with Berries are a nutritious and fluffy pancake dish.

Value of Nutrition

- ✓ 250 kcal of calories
- ✓ 8 g of protein
- ✓ 40 g of carbohydrates
- ✓ 6 g of fat
- ✓ 6 g of fiber

Jordan Marguire

Ingredients:

- ✓ One cup flour made from whole grains
- ✓ Dollop of baking powder
- ✓ One tablespoon sugar (optional) or sweetness
- ✓ One egg
- ✓ One cup of milk or a nondairy substitute
- ✓ Two tsp melted oil or butter
- ✓ Topping: fresh berries

Steps in Meal Preparations:

- ✓ Combine whole grain flour, baking powder, and sugar (if desired) in a bowl.
- ✓ Whisk the egg, milk, and melted butter or oil in a separate basin.
- ✓ Mix the dry and wet components together, being careful not to overmix.
- ✓ Heat a griddle or pan that has been gently greased over medium heat.
- ✓ For each pancake, transfer 1/4 cup of batter to the skillet.

✓ Cook until surface bubbles appear, then turn and continue cooking until golden brown

✓ Present pancakes with fresh berries on top.

Why Seniors Can Benefit from It:

✓ Benefits of Whole Grains: Seniors' heart health and digestion are improved by the extra minerals and fiber that whole grain flour offers.

✓ Antioxidant-Rich Berries: Packed with vitamins and antioxidants, berries help seniors' immune systems and brain function.

✓ Easy to Digest: Seniors with dietary restrictions can enjoy these whole grain pancakes as they are less taxing on the digestive tract.

Roasted Pork Tenderloin with Garlic Herbs

Tender and juicy pork is produced by roasting garlic and herbs to perfection in this tasty meal called Garlic Herb Roasted Pork Tenderloin.

Jordan Marguire

Value of Nutrition

- ✓ 280 kcal of calories
- ✓ 30 g of protein
- ✓ Two grams of carbohydrates
- ✓ 16 grams of fat
- ✓ Fiber: 0

Ingredients:

- ✓ One tenderloin of pork
- ✓ four minced garlic cloves
- ✓ Fresh herbs, such as sage, thyme, or rosemary
- ✓ To taste, add salt and pepper.
- ✓ Olive oil

- ✓ Steps in Meal Preparation:
- ✓ Turn the oven on to 375°F, or 190°C.
- ✓ Add salt, pepper, minced garlic, and chopped fresh herbs to the pork tenderloin.
- ✓ Melt the olive oil in a pan over medium-high heat.
- ✓ Until browned, sear the pork on both sides.

- ✓ Spoon the pork onto a baking tray and bake until the internal temperature reaches 145°F (63°C), 25 to 30 minutes.
- ✓ Before slicing and serving, give it a few minutes of resting.

Why Seniors Can Benefit from It:

- ✓ High-quality Protein: As a lean protein source, pork tenderloin helps older people maintain their muscles.
- ✓ Herbs and Spices: Antioxidants and anti-inflammatory qualities found in garlic and herbs improve general health in the elderly.
- ✓ Soft Texture: Pork tenderloin has a soft texture that is simpler for seniors to chew and digest when cooked correctly.

Lettuce Wraps Taco Style

Taco Lettuce Wraps are a healthier take on classic tacos, made with seasoned meat, veggies, and toppings inside a crispy shell made of lettuce leaves.

Jordan Marguire

Value of Nutrition

- ✓ 220 kcal of calories
- ✓ 18 g of protein
- ✓ 10grams of carbohydrates
- ✓ 12 grams of fat
- ✓ 4 g of fiber

Ingredients:

- ✓ 1 pound of ground turkey or beef
- ✓ Mixture for taco seasoning
- ✓ lettuce leaves (romaine or iceberg)
- ✓ chopped tomatoes
- ✓ Cheese in shredded form
- ✓ sour cream (not required)
- ✓ Avocado slices (optional)

Steps in Meal Preparation:

- ✓ Over medium heat, brown ground beef or turkey in a pan.
- ✓ After removing any extra fat, add the taco seasoning mix as directed on the container.

- ✓ The meat should be nicely covered and seasoned after a few minutes of simmering.
- ✓ To prepare lettuce leaves for stuffing, wash and separate them.
- ✓ Top each lettuce cup with the seasoned meat, shredded cheese, chopped tomatoes, and any additional toppings you like.
- ✓ Serve Taco Lettuce Wraps with avocado slices or sour cream if desired.

Why Seniors Can Benefit from It:

- ✓ Protein Source: The essential protein for the health and regeneration of elderly muscles is found in ground beef or turkey.
- ✓ Low-Carb Option: Since lettuce contains fewer carbs than tortillas, it is a good choice for seniors who are managing their carb consumption.
- ✓ Tailorable and Simple to Consume: Lettuce wraps provide seniors with a customisable, bite-sized meal that is simple to put together.

Glazed Carrots in Orange

Orange Glazed Carrots are a delicious side dish made of soft carrots covered in a sweet and tart orange sauce.

Value of Nutrition

- ✓ 90 kcal of calories
- ✓ One gram of protein
- ✓ 20 g of carbohydrates
- ✓ 0.5 g of fat
- ✓ 4 g of fiber

Ingredients:

- ✓ One pound of peeled and sliced carrots
- ✓ Two teaspoons of olive oil or butter
- ✓ Half a cup of orange juice
- ✓ One orange's zest
- ✓ Two teaspoons of maple syrup or honey
- ✓ To taste, add salt and pepper.
- ✓ Parsley, chopped (optional; as a garnish)

Steps in Meal Preparation:

✓ Sliced carrots should be added to boiling water in a pot. Cook until they become crisp-tender, about 5 to 7 minutes. After draining, set away.

✓ Melt butter or warm up olive oil in the same pot over medium heat.

✓ Add the orange zest and juice, salt, pepper, honey or maple syrup. Mix well until fully incorporated.

✓ When the carrots are caramelized and the sauce thickens, add the cooked carrots to the pot and simmer, stirring periodically, for five to seven minutes.

✓ If preferred, top the orange-glazed carrots with minced parsley.

Why Seniors Can Benefit from It:

✓ Rich in Antioxidants: Beta-carotene from carrots and vitamin C from oranges enhance the health of seniors' immune systems and eyes.

- ✓ Low-Calorie Side Dish: This dish adds flavor and nutrition to senior meals while being low in calories and providing a hint of natural sweetness.
- ✓ simple to Chew and Digest: Cooked carrots are a great option for seniors who might have trouble with harsher textures because they are soft and simple to chew.

Kebabs with tofu and vegetables

Tofu & Vegetable Kebabs are tasty and nourishing skewers of marinated tofu and a variety of vegetables that are cooked to perfection on a grill.

Value of Nutrition

- ✓ 180 kcal of calories
- ✓ 12 g of protein
- ✓ 15 g of carbohydrates
- ✓ 8 g of fat
- ✓ 5 g of fiber

Ingredients:

- ✓ One block of pressed and diced extra-firm tofu
- ✓ Various veggies, including onions, bell peppers, cherry tomatoes, and zucchini
- ✓ Regarding the marinade:
- ✓ Two tsp soy sauce
- ✓ Two tsp olive oil
- ✓ two minced garlic cloves
- ✓ One tsp honey or maple syrup
- ✓ one tsp finely chopped ginger
- ✓ To taste, add salt and pepper.

Steps in Meal Preparation:

- ✓ Turn the heat up to medium-high on the grill or grill pan.
- ✓ Combine the marinade ingredients in a bowl.
- ✓ Alternately thread skewers with mixed veggies and pieces of tofu.
- ✓ Apply a thick coating of marinade to the kebabs.

✓ The kebabs should be cooked for ten to twelve minutes, rotating them once, or until the tofu is gently browned and the veggies are soft.

✓ Serve the heated tofu and vegetable kebabs with chopped herbs as a garnish, if desired.

Why Seniors Can Benefit from It:

✓ Plant-Based Protein: Tofu is an excellent source of plant-based protein that helps seniors maintain their general health and muscular mass.

✓ Rich in Nutrients: A variety of vitamins, minerals, and antioxidants found in different vegetables promote the health of elders.

✓ Easy-to-Eat Option: After grilling, the veggies and tofu become softer, which makes them simpler for seniors to chew and process.

Baked Apples with Cinnamon

Warm cinnamon tastes are infused into soft baked apples to create a soothing dessert or snack known as Baked Apples with Cinnamon.

Value of Nutrition

- ✓ 120 kcal of calories
- ✓ One gram of protein
- ✓ 30 g of carbohydrates
- ✓ 0.5 g of fat
- ✓ 5 g of fiber

Ingredients:

- ✓ 4 apples, cut in half and cored
- ✓ Two teaspoons of coconut oil or melted butter
- ✓ Two teaspoons of brown sugar or your preferred sweetness
- ✓ one tsp finely ground cinnamon
- ✓ Optional garnishes include chopped almonds, raisins, or a honey drizzle.

Jordan Marguire

Steps in Meal Preparation:

✓ Turn the oven on to 375°F, or 190°C.

✓ Brown sugar, ground cinnamon, and melted butter or coconut oil should all be combined in a bowl.

✓ Put the cored and cut apples on a baking sheet or a tray covered with parchment paper.

✓ Make sure the apple halves are well covered by brushing them with the cinnamon mixture.

✓ Bake the apples for 20 to 25 minutes, or until they are soft and starting to caramelize slightly.

✓ If preferred, top baked apples with optional toppings.

Why Seniors Can Benefit from It:

✓ High Fiber Content: Apples are a wonderful source of fiber, which helps seniors' hearts and aids with digestion.

✓ Antioxidant Characteristics: Cinnamon is well-known for having antioxidant characteristics that may improve general health in seniors.

✓ Soft Texture: As baked apples simmer, they become softer, making them a great, simple-to-eat treat for older adults.

Brown rice, chicken, and vegetable stir-fried

This recipe, called Chicken and Vegetable Stir-Fry with Brown Rice, is a vibrant and aromatic combination of perfectly stir-fried delicate chicken, a variety of veggies, and nutty brown rice.

Value of Nutrition

✓ 320 kcal of calories

✓ 25 g of protein

✓ 35 g of carbohydrates

✓ 8 g of fat

✓ 6 g of fiber

Ingredients:

✓ Two breasts of chicken, cut into strips

Jordan Marguire

- ✓ Two cups of mixed veggies, including snap peas, broccoli, carrots, and bell peppers
- ✓ Two minced garlic cloves
- ✓ One tablespoon of finely chopped ginger
- ✓ Three tsp low-sodium soybean sauce
- ✓ One tablespoon of sesame oil
- ✓ Brown rice cooked and ready to serve

Steps in Meal Preparation:

- ✓ In a large skillet or wok, heat the sesame oil over medium-high heat.
- ✓ Stir in the grated ginger and minced garlic for 30 seconds, or until fragrant.
- ✓ Cook the chicken strips until they are well cooked and browned.
- ✓ Add the mixed veggies and stir-fry them until they become crisp and tender.
- ✓ Stir to blend with low-sodium soy sauce before adding it to the mixture.
- ✓ Over cooked brown rice, serve the stir-fried chicken and vegetables.

Why Seniors Can Benefit from It:

✓ Lean Protein Source: Chicken provides seniors with high-quality protein that is necessary for muscle growth and repair.

✓ Vegetables Rich in Nutrients: A variety of vegetables include vitamins, minerals, and antioxidants that promote the health of older citizens.

✓ Fiber-Rich Brown Rice: Brown rice is a high-fiber carbohydrate that helps seniors' blood sugar levels stay stable and aids in digestion.

Roasted Herb Vegetables

Herb-Roasted Vegetables are a tasty and nourishing side dish made from a colorful blend of seasonal vegetables roasted with aromatic herbs.

Value of Nutrition:

✓ 120 kcal of calories

✓ 3 g of protein

✓ 15 g of carbohydrates

Jordan Marguire

- ✓ 6 g of fat
- ✓ 5 g of fiber

Ingredients:
- ✓ A variety of veggies, such as Brussels sprouts, cauliflower, bell peppers, and carrots
- ✓ Two tsp olive oil
- ✓ Two tsp mixed dry herbs (oregano, thyme, and rosemary)
- ✓ To taste, add salt and pepper.

Steps in Meal Preparation:
- ✓ Set the oven temperature to 425°F (220°C).
- ✓ Prepare and dice a variety of veggies into pieces of comparable size.
- ✓ Toss the veggies in a big basin with salt, pepper, olive oil, and mixed dried herbs until they are well covered.
- ✓ Arrange the veggies on a baking pan so they are in a single layer.

- ✓ Roast for 20 to 25 minutes, or until the veggies are soft and starting to caramelize, in a preheated oven.
- ✓ Warm herb-roasted veggies make a delicious side dish.

Why Seniors Can Benefit from It:

- ✓ Nutrient-Rich Content: A range of vitamins, minerals, and antioxidants are included in mixed veggies, which support general health in older adults.
- ✓ Vegetables that have been roasted enhance their inherent sweetness and become softer, which facilitates simpler digestion for elderly people.
- ✓ Flexible and Customizable: Seniors' dietary requirements and tastes may be met with this recipe's ability to work with a variety of veggies.

Smoothie with peanut butter and bananas

A healthful treat, the Peanut Butter and Banana Smoothie combines creamy peanut butter, ripe bananas, and dairy or non-dairy milk into a smooth and pleasant drink.

Value of Nutrition

- ✓ 280 kcal of calories
- ✓ 12 g of protein
- ✓ 30 g of carbohydrates
- ✓ 14 grams of fat
- ✓ 6 g of fiber

Ingredients:

- ✓ Two ripe bananas, cut into slices and peeled
- ✓ Two teaspoons of unsweetened peanut butter
- ✓ One cup of milk or a nondairy substitute
- ✓ One tablespoon of optional sweetener, such as honey
- ✓ Cubes of ice (optional)

Steps in Meal Preparation:

Jordan Marguire

- ✓ In a blender, combine peanut butter, milk (or a plant-based substitute), sliced bananas, and honey (if desired).
- ✓ If you want your smoothie cooler, add some ice cubes.
- ✓ Blend till creamy and smooth.
- ✓ Serve the Peanut Butter and Banana Smoothie right away after pouring it into a glass.

Why Seniors Can Benefit from It:

- ✓ Protein and Energy Source: Natural carbohydrates and protein are found in peanut butter and bananas, which provide seniors energy.
- ✓ Simple to Consume: Smoothies are a simple method for seniors to acquire critical nutrients, especially if they have trouble eating solid foods. They are also easy to drink.
- ✓ Rich in Nutrients: Seniors' general well-being is enhanced by the abundance of vitamins, minerals, and healthy fats in this smoothie.

Casserole of Cabbage Rolls

Baked to perfection, Cabbage Roll Casserole is a deconstructed version of the traditional cabbage roll, made with ground beef, rice, cabbage, and tomato sauce.

Value of Nutrition:

- ✓ 290 kcal of calories
- ✓ 18 g of protein
- ✓ 25 g of carbohydrates
- ✓ 12 grams of fat
- ✓ 6 g of fiber

Ingredients:

- ✓ 1 pound of ground turkey or beef
- ✓ One chopped onion
- ✓ two minced garlic cloves
- ✓ one head of finely chopped cabbage
- ✓ one cup of rice, cooked
- ✓ One 14-oz can of tomato sauce
- ✓ One 14-oz can of chopped tomatoes

- ✓ To taste, add salt and pepper.
- ✓ Cheese shreds, if desired, for topping

Steps in Meal Preparation:

- ✓ Turn the oven on to 375°F, or 190°C.
- ✓ Over medium heat, cook ground beef or turkey in a large pan.
- ✓ Cook the minced garlic and chopped onions together until the onions become transparent.
- ✓ Add chopped cabbage and simmer, stirring, until just starting to soften.
- ✓ Add the diced tomatoes, tomato sauce, cooked rice, salt, and pepper. Blend well.
- ✓ Spread the mixture evenly in a baking dish after transferring it there.
- ✓ Add some shredded cheese on top if you'd like.
- ✓ Bake for 25 to 30 minutes, or until the top is golden brown and bubbling.
- ✓ Warm up the casserole with cabbage rolls.

Why Seniors Can Benefit from It:

✓ Protein and Fiber Content: The protein and fiber in ground pork and cabbage help seniors' digestion and general health.

✓ One-Pan dinner: This casserole simplifies dinner preparation and cleanup for seniors by providing a range of nutrients in a single dish.

✓ Flavorful and Comforting: For seniors seeking comfort food, Cabbage Roll Casserole provides flavors reminiscent of classic cabbage rolls.

Halibut baked with herbs and lemon

A light and delectable fish lunch, Baked Halibut with Lemon and Herbs is a lovely dish made with soft halibut fillets baked with zesty lemon and savory herbs.

Value of Nutrition

✓ 180 kcal of calories

✓ 30 g of protein

✓ Two grams of carbohydrates

Jordan Marguire

- ✓ 5 grams of fat
- ✓ Fiber: 0

Ingredients:

- ✓ Four fillets of halibut
- ✓ Two tsp olive oil
- ✓ One lemon's juice
- ✓ One lemon's zest
- ✓ Two minced garlic cloves
- ✓ Fresh herbs, such thyme, dill, or parsley
- ✓ To taste, add salt and pepper.

Steps in Meal Preparation:

- ✓ Turn the oven on to 375°F, or 190°C.
- ✓ Fish fillets should be put on a baking dish.
- ✓ Olive oil, lemon juice, zest, minced garlic, chopped fresh herbs, salt, and pepper should all be combined in a small basin.
- ✓ Make sure the halibut fillets are uniformly covered by pouring the liquid over them.

- ✓ Fish should flake easily with a fork and be cooked through after 12 to 15 minutes in the oven.
- ✓ If preferred, top the hot baked halibut with lemon and herbs with more herbs.

Why Seniors Can Benefit from It:

- ✓ High-quality Protein: Seniors' muscular strength and restoration depend on the high-protein content of halibut, a lean fish.
- ✓ Omega-3 Fatty Acids: Omega-3s, which are found in fish like halibut, help seniors' hearts and brains.
- ✓ Light and Digestible: For seniors seeking a tasty, light supper, baked fish is a good choice because it is typically simple to digest.

Goat cheese salad with beets

This salad of roasted beets, creamy goat cheese, crunchy almonds, and crisp greens is served with a zesty vinaigrette, creating a delightful and reviving combination.

Jordan Marguire

Value of Nutrition

- ✓ 220 kcal of calories
- ✓ 8 g of protein
- ✓ 15 g of carbohydrates
- ✓ 16 grams of fat
- ✓ 4 g of fiber

Ingredients:

- ✓ Two to three medium-sized beets, sliced and roasted
- ✓ Four cups of mixed salad greens, such as mixed greens, arugula, or spinach
- ✓ 2 oz of crumbled goat cheese
- ✓ 1/4 cup chopped, roasted walnuts or pecans
- ✓ For the salad dressing:
- ✓ Half a tsp balsamic vinegar
- ✓ one-fourth cup olive oil
- ✓ One tsp Dijon mustard
- ✓ To taste, add salt and pepper.

Jordan Marguire

Steps in Meal Preparation:

✓ Turn the oven on to 400°F, or 200°C. Cover beets with foil and roast until soft, 45 to 60 minutes. After letting cool, peel and cut.

✓ To create the vinaigrette, combine the olive oil, Dijon mustard, balsamic vinegar, salt, and pepper in a small bowl.

✓ Combine the mixed salad greens with half of the vinaigrette in a big bowl.

✓ Place the dressed greens onto a platter for presentation. Add toasted nuts, crumbled goat cheese, and roasted beet slices on top.

✓ Serve the salad with the leftover vinaigrette drizzled over it or on the side.

Why Seniors Can Benefit from It:

✓ Nutrient-Rich Beets: Rich in vitamins, minerals, and antioxidants, beets promote the immune system and general health of seniors.

✓ Goat cheese is a good source of calcium, which is necessary for healthy bones in older people.

✓ Heart-Healthy Greens: Mixed salad greens help with digestion and support heart health since they are high in fiber and vitamins.

Salmon with a Honey Mustard Glaze

A tasty and nutrient-dense dish, Honey Mustard Glazed Salmon is made with delicate salmon fillets covered in a sweet and spicy glaze.

Value of Nutrition

✓ 280 kcal of calories

✓ 22 g of protein

✓ Ten grams of carbohydrates

✓ 16 grams of fat

✓ 0.5 g of fiber

Ingredients:

✓ Four fillets of salmon

✓ Two tsp honey

✓ Two tsp Dijon mustard

Jordan Marguire

- ✓ One tablespoon of olive oil
- ✓ Two minced garlic cloves
- ✓ To taste, add salt and pepper.
- ✓ Fresh herbs for garnish, such as dill or parsley

Steps in Meal Preparation

- ✓ Turn the oven on to 400°F, or 200°C.
- ✓ Combine the honey, Dijon mustard, olive oil, minced garlic, salt, and pepper in a bowl.
- ✓ Arrange the salmon fillets on a parchment paper-lined baking pan.
- ✓ Dredge the salmon fillets in a thick layer of the honey mustard mixture.
- ✓ Bake the salmon for 12 to 15 minutes, or until it is cooked through and flake readily with a fork.
- ✓ Before serving, garnish the salmon with a honey mustard glaze using fresh herbs.

Why Seniors Can Benefit from It:

- ✓ Omega-3 Fatty Acids: Rich in omega-3s, salmon helps seniors' hearts and brains stay healthy.
- ✓ Protein and Vital Nutrients: High-quality protein and important nutrients are found in salmon, which is beneficial for seniors' general health and wellbeing.
- ✓ Sweet and Easy to Digest: The honey mustard glaze gives this meal a taste that's not only tasty but also simple for seniors to chew and absorb.

Pudding with Chia Seeds

Soaked chia seeds in milk or yogurt, then sweetened and seasoned to taste, Chia Seed Pudding is a creamy, nutrient-dense dessert or breakfast choice.

Value of Nutrition:

- ✓ 180 kcal of calories
- ✓ Six grams of protein
- ✓ 20 g of carbohydrates

Jordan Marguire

✓ 9 g of fat

✓ 12 grams of fiber

Ingredients:

✓ One-fourth cup chia seeds

✓ One cup of milk (almond, coconut, or any other type of milk preferable)

✓ One tablespoon of maple syrup or honey (optional)

✓ Half a teaspoon of extract from vanilla

✓ Toppings: fresh fruits, nuts, or seeds

Steps in Meal Preparation:

✓ Chia seeds, milk, vanilla extract, honey (if used), and maple syrup should all be combined in a bowl. Mix well by stirring.

✓ To enable the chia seeds to absorb the liquid and thicken, cover the bowl and place it in the refrigerator for a minimum of four hours or overnight.

✓ To guarantee a creamy texture, stir the chia seed mixture just before serving.

✓ To enhance taste and texture, garnish Chia Seed Pudding with fresh fruits, nuts, or seeds and serve it in separate bowls or jars.

Why Seniors Can Benefit from It:

✓ Rich in Fiber: Chia seeds have a high fiber content that helps seniors feel full and supports digestive health.

✓ Omega-3 Fatty Acids: Seniors' hearts benefit from the omega-3s found in chia seeds, which also lower inflammation.

✓ Simple Dessert or Breakfast: Chia Seed Pudding is a great choice for elderly people who have trouble chewing or swallowing because it is soft and simple to swallow.

Acorn Squash Stuffed

Roasted acorn squash halves stuffed with a delectable blend of grains, veggies, and savory toppings make for a visually stunning and delectable meal known as stuffed acorn squash.

Value of Nutrition

- ✓ 320 kcal of calories
- ✓ 8 g of protein
- ✓ 60 grams of carbohydrates
- ✓ 6 g of fat
- ✓ Fiber: nine grams

Ingredients:

- ✓ Half two acorn squashes and remove the seeds.
- ✓ One cup cooked rice or quinoa
- ✓ One cup of mixed veggies, such as onions, mushrooms, and bell peppers
- ✓ One can (15 oz) of rinsed and drained black beans
- ✓ One teaspoon of cumin
- ✓ One tsp of paprika
- ✓ To taste, add salt and pepper.
- ✓ Use olive oil to drizzle
- ✓ For garnish, use fresh herbs (optional).

Steps in Meal Preparation

- ✓ Turn the oven on to 375°F, or 190°C.
- ✓ Half the acorn squash and place it cut-side up on a baking pan. Add a drizzle of olive oil and season with pepper and salt.
- ✓ Bake the squash for 25 to 30 minutes, or until they are soft when pierced with a fork.
- ✓ Sauté mixed veggies in a pan until they are soft. Add the black beans, cumin, paprika, cooked rice or quinoa, salt, and pepper. Blend well.
- ✓ Stuff the quinoa and veggie mixture into the baked halves of the acorn squash.
- ✓ Place the filled squash back in the oven and let it roast for ten or fifteen more minutes.
- ✓ Before serving, add a fresh herb garnish.

Why Seniors Can Benefit from It:

- ✓ High Fiber and Nutrient Content: Mixed veggies and acorn squash offer vital nutrients and dietary fiber, which improves digestion and enhances general health in older adults.

- ✓ Versatile and Customizable: The filling is adaptable to dietary choices and may be tailored to meet a range of senior nutritional demands.
- ✓ Delicate Texture: Tenderized by roasting, roasted acorn squash has a delicate texture that makes it simple for seniors to chew and assimilate.

Turkey and Bean Chili Recipe

A filling and healthy recipe, Turkey and Bean Chili is a robust and savory concoction of lean ground turkey, beans, veggies, and fragrant spices.

Value of Nutrition:

- ✓ 280 kcal of calories
- ✓ 22 g of protein
- ✓ 30 g of carbohydrates
- ✓ 8 g of fat
- ✓ Ten grams of fiber

Jordan Marguire

Ingredients:
- ✓ One pound of ground turkey
- ✓ One chopped onion
- ✓ Two minced garlic cloves
- ✓ One can (15 oz) of washed and drained kidney beans
- ✓ One can (15 oz) of rinsed and drained black beans
- ✓ One 14-oz can of chopped tomatoes
- ✓ Two cups chicken broth reduced in sodium
- ✓ Two tsp of chili powder
- ✓ One teaspoon of cumin
- ✓ To taste, add salt and pepper.
- ✓ Topping options include chopped cilantro, sour cream, and shredded cheese.

Steps in Meal Preparation:
- ✓ Cook the ground turkey over medium heat in a big saucepan or Dutch oven until browned.
- ✓ Cook the chopped onion and minced garlic together until the onions become transparent.

- ✓ Add the diced tomatoes, kidney and black beans, chicken broth, cumin, chili powder, salt, and pepper and stir.
- ✓ After bringing the chili to a boil, lower the heat and simmer it for twenty to twenty-five minutes to let the flavors combine.
- ✓ Serve the Turkey and Bean Chili hot, garnished with extras if you'd like. Adjust spice as necessary.

Why Seniors Can Benefit from It:

- ✓ Lean Protein Source: Ground turkey provides the lean protein seniors need to maintain and strengthen their muscles.
- ✓ High Fiber Content: Seniors who eat beans might feel fuller and have better digestion because to their high fiber content.
- ✓ Vitamins and Minerals: The variety of veggies and spices in this chili provide vital vitamins and minerals that promote seniors' general health.

Barley and Mushroom Soup

The warm and delectable meal of Mushroom Barley Soup is made with soft mushrooms, pearl barley, vegetables, and savory spices. It is a substantial and healthy soup.

Value of Nutrition:

- ✓ 220 kcal of calories
- ✓ 8 g of protein
- ✓ 40 g of carbohydrates
- ✓ 3 g of fat
- ✓ 8 g of fiber

Ingredients:

- ✓ One cup of washed pearl barley
- ✓ Eight cups of chicken or veggie stock
- ✓ Two tsp olive oil
- ✓ One sliced onion
- ✓ Two minced garlic cloves
- ✓ 8 oz of chopped mushrooms

Jordan Marguire

- ✓ Two chopped carrots
- ✓ Two chopped celery stalks
- ✓ One bay leaf
- ✓ To taste, add salt and pepper.
- ✓ Fresh parsley that has been chopped (optional)

Steps in Meal Preparation:

- ✓ Warm up the olive oil in a big saucepan over medium heat. Add the minced garlic and onion, and sauté until aromatic.
- ✓ Add the chopped celery, carrots, and mushrooms. Cook until the veggies start to get tender, about a few minutes.
- ✓ Pour in the chicken or vegetable broth and stir in the washed pearl barley and bay leaf.
- ✓ After bringing the soup to a boil, lower the heat, and simmer it until the barley is soft, 45 to 50 minutes.
- ✓ To taste, add salt and pepper for seasoning. Before serving, take the bay leaf off.
- ✓ If preferred, add some finely chopped fresh parsley to the Mushroom Barley Soup.

Jordan Marguire

Why Seniors Can Benefit from It:

✓ The nutritional value of pearl barley is high in fiber and other elements that are good for the digestive system and general health of seniors.

✓ Health Benefits of Mushrooms: Rich in vitamins and antioxidants, mushrooms may improve the immune and general well-being of seniors.

✓ Easy-to-Digest Soup: For seniors who like readily chewable and digestible meals, this soup's soft texture and vegetable combination are ideal.

Fruit bowl with cottage cheese

A lovely and nutritious snack or breakfast choice, the cottage cheese and fruit bowl is a simple yet fulfilling meal that combines creamy cottage cheese with a selection of fresh fruits.

Value of Nutrition

✓ 220 kcal of calories

Jordan Marguire

- ✓ 15 g of protein
- ✓ 25 g of carbohydrates
- ✓ 8 g of fat
- ✓ 3 g of fiber

Ingredients:
- ✓ One cup cottage cheese, either standard or low-fat
- ✓ A variety of fresh fruits (including peaches, chopped apples, bananas, and berries)
- ✓ Two teaspoons of maple syrup or honey (optional)
- ✓ Nuts or seeds (optional) as garnish

Steps in Meal Preparation:
- ✓ Transfer cottage cheese to a platter.
- ✓ Place your preferred assortment of fresh fruits on top of the cottage cheese.
- ✓ If preferred, drizzle with maple syrup or honey for extra sweetness.
- ✓ Add some nuts or seeds for flavor and texture.

Why Seniors Can Benefit from It:

✓ Rich in Protein: Cottage cheese is a fantastic source of protein, which is necessary for the maintenance and repair of older citizens' muscles.

✓ Vitamins and Minerals from Fruits: Seniors' immune systems and general health are supported by the vitamins, minerals, and antioxidants found in fresh fruits.

✓ Quick and Simple Preparation: This straightforward recipe may be tailored to seniors' dietary requirements and preferred fruits. It is simple to make.

Stir-fried Sesame Ginger Beef

Sesame Ginger Beef Stir-Fry is a savory recipe that combines vibrant veggies, delicate beef strips, and a delectable sesame ginger sauce to create a filling and healthy dinner.

Jordan Marguire

Value of Nutrition

- ✓ 320 kcal of calories
- ✓ 24 g of protein
- ✓ 20 g of carbohydrates
- ✓ 16 grams of fat
- ✓ 4 g of fiber

Ingredients:

- ✓ One pound of finely cut beef sirloin
- ✓ Two tsp of sesame oil
- ✓ Two minced garlic cloves
- ✓ One tablespoon of freshly grated ginger
- ✓ Two cups of mixed veggies, such as carrots, snap peas, broccoli, and bell peppers
- ✓ Three tsp of soy sauce
- ✓ One tablespoon of brown sugar or honey
- ✓ One-tspn rice vinegar
- ✓ Sunflower seeds as a garnish
- ✓ Prepared quinoa or brown rice for serving

Jordan Marguire

Steps in Meal Preparation:

- ✓ To make the sauce, put the soy sauce, rice vinegar, and honey or brown sugar in a bowl. Put aside.
- ✓ In a large skillet or wok, heat the sesame oil over medium-high heat.
- ✓ Add the grated ginger and minced garlic, and cook for one minute, or until fragrant.
- ✓ Stir-fry the thinly sliced meat in the pan until it becomes brown. Take out and put aside the steak from the griddle.
- ✓ Stir-fry mixed veggies in the same skillet until they are the desired softness.
- ✓ Place the steak back into the skillet and cover the meat and veggies with the prepared sauce. Toss to mix thoroughly and coat uniformly.
- ✓ Simmer for one more minute, or until the sauce gradually thickens and envelops the ingredients.
- ✓ Serve the stir-fried sesame ginger beef over cooked quinoa or brown rice, and top with sesame seeds.

Why Seniors Can Benefit from It:

✓ Protein and Nutrient-Dense: Beef is a rich source of protein and vital nutrients that are good for the general health and muscle strength of seniors.

✓ Vibrant and Colorful veggies: The combination of veggies provides seniors with antioxidants, vitamins, and minerals that boost their immune systems.

✓ Simple-to-Eat Stir-Fry: This dish is easy for seniors to chew and digest thanks to the thinly sliced beef and soft veggies.

Pasta with Lemon Garlic Shrimp

This recipe for Lemon Garlic Shrimp Pasta combines savory and filling ingredients such as al dente pasta, succulent shrimp, and a zesty lemon garlic sauce.

Value of Nutrition

✓ 350 kcal of calories

✓ 25 g of protein

✓ 40 g of carbohydrates

Jordan Marguire

✓ Ten grams of fat
✓ 3 g of fiber

Ingredients:

✓ 8 ounces of pasta (spaghetti, linguine, or other favorite kind)
✓ One pound of peeled and deveined shrimp
✓ Two tsp olive oil
✓ Four minced garlic cloves
✓ One lemon's zest
✓ One lemon's juice
✓ Flakes of red pepper (optional)
✓ To taste, add salt and pepper.
✓ Freshly chopped parsley as a garnish

Steps in Meal Preparation

✓ As directed on the package, cook pasta in boiling salted water until it's al dente. After draining, set away.
✓ Heat the olive oil in a big skillet over medium heat.

- ✓ Garlic powder should be added to the skillet and cooked for 30 seconds or less, or until aromatic.
- ✓ Add the shrimp to the skillet and cook for 2 to 3 minutes on each side, or until they are pink and opaque.
- ✓ Add the lemon juice, zest, and red pepper flakes (if using) and stir. Add pepper and salt for seasoning.
- ✓ When the pasta is ready, add it to the skillet with the shrimp and toss to thoroughly heat everything.
- ✓ Garnish the hot Lemon Garlic Shrimp Pasta with finely chopped fresh parsley.

Why Seniors Can Benefit from It:

- ✓ High-quality Protein: Lean protein, such that found in shrimp, is essential for seniors' muscles to be strengthened and repaired.
- ✓ Light and tasty Dish: For seniors seeking a filling dinner, this pasta dish is tasty yet still simple to chew and assimilate.

✓ Vitamin C from Lemon: Vitamin C from lemons supports the immune systems and general health of elders..

30 DAYS MEAL PLAN

Day 1

Breakfast: Greek Yogurt Parfait

Lunch: Spinach with Feta Stuffed Chicken Breast

Dinner: Roasted Vegetable Soup

Day 2

Breakfast: Whole Grain Pancakes with Berries

Lunch: Lentil and Vegetable Curry

Dinner: Baked Halibut with Herbs and Lemon

Day 3

Breakfast: Cottage Cheese and Fruit Bowl

Lunch: Rainbow Veggie Wraps

Dinner: Sesame Ginger Beef Stir-Fry

Day 4

Breakfast: Chia Seed Pudding

Lunch: Turkey and Bean Chili

Dinner: Ratatouille

Day 5

Breakfast: Whole Grain Pancakes with Berries

Lunch: Mushroom Barley Soup

Dinner: Lemon Garlic Shrimp Pasta

Day 6

Breakfast: Coconut Curry Shrimp

Lunch: Cabbage Roll Casserole

Dinner: Stuffed Acorn Squash

Day 7

Breakfast: Greek Yogurt Parfait

Lunch: Sesame Ginger Beef Stir-Fry

Dinner: Beet and Goat Cheese Salad

Week 2:

Day 8

Breakfast: Stuffed Acorn Squash

Lunch: Honey Mustard Glazed Salmon

Dinner: Baked Cod with Herbs

Day 9

Breakfast: Cottage Cheese and Fruit Bowl

Lunch: Chickpea and Spinach Curry

Dinner: Taco Lettuce Wraps

Day 10

Breakfast: Whole Grain Pancakes with Berries

Lunch: Beet and Goat Cheese Salad

Dinner: Garlic Herb Roasted Pork Tenderloin

Day 11

Breakfast: Chia Seed Pudding

Lunch: Sesame Ginger Tofu Stir-Fry

Dinner: Chicken and Vegetable Stir-Fry with Brown Rice

Day 12

Breakfast: Greek Yogurt Parfait

Lunch: Mushroom Barley Soup

Dinner: Roasted Vegetable Soup

Day 13

Breakfast: Coconut Curry Shrimp

Lunch: Baked Sweet Potato Fries

Dinner: Caprese Salad

Day 14

Breakfast: Cottage Cheese and Fruit Bowl

Lunch: Lemon Garlic Shrimp Pasta

Dinner: Stuffed Portobello Mushrooms

Week 3:

Day 15

Breakfast: Chia Seed Pudding

Lunch: Sesame Ginger Tofu Stir-Fry

Dinner: Garlic Herb Roasted Pork Tenderloin

Day 16

Breakfast: Greek Yogurt Parfait

Lunch: Beet and Goat Cheese Salad

Dinner: Roasted Vegetable Soup

Day 17

Breakfast: Cottage Cheese and Fruit Bowl

Lunch: Mushroom Barley Soup

Dinner: Chicken and Vegetable Stir-Fry with Brown Rice

Day 18

Breakfast: Coconut Curry Shrimp

Lunch: Baked Sweet Potato Fries

Dinner: Caprese Salad

Day 19

Breakfast: Cottage Cheese and Fruit Bowl

Lunch: Lemon Garlic Shrimp Pasta

Dinner: Stuffed Portobello Mushrooms

Day 20

Breakfast: Whole Grain Pancakes with Berries

Lunch: Ratatouille

Dinner: Orange Glazed Carrots

Day 21

Breakfast: Greek Yogurt Parfait

Lunch: Taco Lettuce Wraps

Dinner: Honey Mustard Glazed Salmon

Week 4:

Day 22

Breakfast: Stuffed Acorn Squash

Lunch: Sesame Ginger Beef Stir-Fry

Dinner: Roasted Vegetable Soup

Day 23

Breakfast: Cottage Cheese and Fruit Bowl

Lunch: Beet and Goat Cheese Salad

Dinner: Baked Halibut with Lemon and Herbs

Day 24

Breakfast: Chia Seed Pudding

Lunch: Chicken and Vegetable Stir-Fry with Brown Rice

Dinner: Lemon Garlic Shrimp Pasta

Day 25

Breakfast: Coconut Curry Shrimp

Lunch: Mushroom Barley Soup

Dinner: Dinner: Ratatouille

Day 26

Breakfast: Cottage Cheese and Fruit Bowl

Lunch: Caprese Salad

Dinner: Honey Mustard Glazed Salmon

Day 27

Breakfast: Greek Yogurt Parfait

Lunch: Stuffed Portobello Mushrooms

Dinner: Taco Lettuce Wraps

Day 28

Breakfast: Whole Grain Pancakes with Berries

Lunch: Orange Glazed Carrots

Dinner: Sesame Ginger Tofu Stir-Fry

Week 5:

Day 29

Breakfast: Lemon Garlic Shrimp Pasta

Lunch: Ratatouille

Dinner: Honey Mustard Glazed Salmon

Day 30

Breakfast: Cottage Cheese and Fruit Bowl

Lunch: Baked Halibut with Lemon and Herbs

Dinner: Stuffed Acorn Squash

This 30-day extended meal plan includes a variety of dishes that follow the DASH diet guidelines and provides a wide selection of wholesome meals. Adapt ingredient and quantity proportions to suit dietary requirements and personal tastes. For individualized nutritional advice, as always, speak with a medical expert or a qualified dietitian, particularly for elderly people or those with certain health issues.

CONCLUSON

The ground-breaking book "The Dash Diet Meal Prep Plan for Seniors: Recipes for Blood Sugar and Boost Energy" transforms the way elders eat healthily. This book is skillfully designed to meet the unique dietary requirements of senior citizens, with an emphasis on blood sugar regulation and energy enhancement. It presents the DASH diet to readers, an extensively studied dietary regimen that is well-known for its ability to control blood pressure and improve heart health in general. The book is unique in that it provides simple meal prep recipes that make eating a healthy diet easier. Every dish has been painstakingly created to be senior-friendly, complete with step-by-step directions and helpful meal planning advice. Healthy eating is made to taste great with these dishes, which range from filling meals to robust breakfasts. They are full of flavor and healthful ingredients.

Do well to drop a review telling us what recipes you enjoyed, or overall, what you enjoyed about this book

Jordan Marguire

and in what areas you would like us to improve in your editions. Thank you!

Jordan Marguire

JOTTINGS

JOTTINGS

Jordan Marguire

JOTTINGS